I0413538

Colon Cleanses to Lose Weight Do They Really Work

Richard C.H. Yates Sr.

This is a 22 chapter guyed for colon cleansing and weight lose

Important Legal Disclaimer

The information in this book reflects the author's opinions and is not intended to replace any medical advice. Before beginning this or any nutritional or exercise regimen, consult your physician first to be sure it is appropriate for you. If you are unsure of any foods recommended, you should always consult your physician's advice. The author has made every effort to supply accurate information in the creation of this book. The author offers no warranty and accepts no responsibility for any loss or damages of any kind that may be incurred by the reader it's a result of action arising from the use of the content in this book.

The reader assumes all responsibility for the use of the information in this text.

Table of Content

Colon Cleanses to Lose Weight: Do They Really Work?

Are you looking to lose weight? If you are, you may have used the internet to research weight loss products. When many of us think of weight loss product, diet pill are often the first thing that comes to mind.

While diet pills may be able to help you achieve your weight loss goals, diet pills are not the only weight loss product that you may want to look into.

A large number of individuals have successfully used colon cleanses, also commonly referred to as weight loss cleanses, to lose weight and you may want to think about doing the same.

When it comes to using colon cleanses to lose weight, there are many individuals, possibly just like you, who wonder how the whole process works. Before understanding how colon cleanses may help you lose weight, it is important to remember that there may be a variance.

There are some colon cleanses that advertise that they are designed to help you lose weight. These types of colon cleanses are also commonly referred to as weight loss cleanses.

With that in mind, there are colon cleanses that advertise that they are not guaranteed to help you lose weight, even though some of them may.

When using a colon cleanse, it is important that you follow all of the instructions given to you. For instance, there are some colon cleanses that require that you do not eat anything for one or two days. These types of colon cleanses are often ones that are in liquid format. The colon cleanses in pill format may request that you only eat and drink certain products, like fruits and vegetables.

If you buy a colon cleanse that asks to you restrict your diet, you are advised to do so. This diet restriction is what makes it possible for you to lose weight, as well as allow the colon cleanse to properly work.

When you use a colon cleanse, you are essentially detoxifying, your body. The colon cleanse will work to push toxins out from your colon and sometimes even your intestines.

This is not only ideal to promote a healthy wellbeing, but it can also help you lose weight. It has been said that the average person has anywhere from four to eight pounds of stored waste in their body.

When using a colon cleanse, that extra waste will be expelled from your body. This is why many individuals are able to lose weight with a colon cleansing.

If you are able to use a rapid colon cleanse, like one that works in three to seven days, you may notice a rapid weight loss. There are some individuals who use colon cleanses to quickly lose weight before a special event like a wedding or a vacation.

While you may be able to achieve rapid weight loss with a colon cleanse, it is important that you proceed with caution.

If you do not change the way that you eat or add exercise to your daily activities, you may see your weight add back on it as little as a few weeks or a few days. This typically happens if you were asked to restrict your diet when using a colon cleanse. While you do not have to keep up with your restricted diet, you are advised to reduce your junk food intake and start a daily or at least a weekly exercise program.

Since it is more than possible for you to lose weight with a colon cleanse, you may be interested in giving one a try. When looking to buy a colon cleanse, you may be able to find them available for sale in traditional department stores, fitness stores, and health stores, both on and offline.

Before buying a colon cleanse, you may want to search for product reviews online or speak with a healthcare professional. This will help to ensure that you if you do buy a colon cleanse that your money is well spent.

Do You Need to Lose Weight? Signs That You May

Each day in the United States, millions of Americans say "I need to lose weight." Are you one of those individuals? While many of the individuals who tell themselves that they need to lose weight do need to lose weight, not all do.

So, the question that many ask themselves is "do I really need to lose weight?" If that is a question that you have asked yourself before, you will want to continue reading on.

One of the many signs that you may need to lose weight is if you are obese. Many individuals do not realize that there is a difference between being overweight and being obese.

While different healthcare professionals have different definitions for obese, it is often said that those who are thirty or forty pounds overweight are obese.

If you are obese, you shouldn't only be worried about your appearance, but your health as well. Obesity has been linked to multiple health complications, including the early onset of death.

Another one of the many signs that you should lose weight is if you have been told that you need to do so. Whether your physician recommended losing weight or if someone that you know on a personal level has, it is advised that you at least take their suggestions into consideration.

Unfortunately, many individuals are embarrassed or become upset when they are told that they need to lose weight.

What you need to remember is that the individual mentioning your weight to you likely isn't as concerned with your appearance as they are with your health.

Another sign that you may want to think about losing weight is if you are finding that your clothes no longer fit you. Of course, it is normal for some individuals to gain weight or to have their weight fluctuate, but you may want to think about joining a weight loss program or developing your own weight loss plan if you find that your clothes no longer fit or are difficult to get into. Unfortunately, many individuals do not just have a small weight gain. Small weight gain often leads to more, which could have a negative impact on your health. It is also important to mention the cost of new clothes, which you may not be able to afford.

If you find many simple tasks or activities, like walking up a flight of stairs, difficult, you may want to think about losing weight. Of course, becoming out of breath from simple activities may not necessarily just be a weight problem, but there is a good chance that it is.

When you lose weight, even just a little bit of it, you will likely find it easier to do many of the activities that you love or even the tasks that you need to do, like take your kids to the park.

The above mentioned signs are just a few of the many signs that you may need to lose weight. Should you wish to lose weight, you are advised to proceed with caution.

There are a number of weight loss products on the market, like diet pills or exercise equipment, which do not work.

To save yourself money and to protect your health, you may want to consider consulting with your physician before starting any weight loss program, even one that you develop yourself.

Fast Weight Loss Tips

Are you interested in losing weight? If you are, are you in a hurry to do so? While it is advised that you do not rely heavily on fast weight loss, also commonly referred to as rapid weight loss, there are many individuals who do.

If you are interested in losing weight, as quickly as possible, you will want to continue reading on.

One of the many ways that you can go about achieving a fat weight loss or rapid weight loss is by reducing the foods that you eat. When reducing your food consumption, it is important that you only reduce your consumption a little bit.

Unfortunately, many individuals who want to achieve fast weight loss think that they need to stop eating altogether, even if it is for two or three days. That is something that you do not want to do.

Once you resume eating again, you will likely gain all of your weight back, almost automatically. It is also important to mention that starving yourself is dangerous to your health.

In conjunction with reducing your food intake, it is advised that you reduce the amount of sweets or junk food that you eat. For fast weight loss, you will want to completely eliminate junk food from your diet, even if it is only for a short period of time.

This means that if you want a snack, you should grab an apple or an orange instead of a chocolate bar or a bag of chips. With candy and other sweets being high in calories, you may see a significant decrease in your calorie consumption by eliminating them from your diet.

Exercise is another way that you can go about achieving fast weight loss. The thing about using exercise to achieve fast weight loss is that it is a little bit tricky.

With exercise, you may not notice a significant weight loss right away. For instance, it typically takes most individuals at least a week or two to notice an improvement in their appearance with the use of exercise.

With that in mind, the more overweight you are, the sooner you may see a decrease in your weight, often quickly.

In keeping with exercise to lose weight, exercise is important to losing weight, as it helps to limit your calorie intake. When you burn off calories, with the use of exercise, your body absorbs fewer calories.

This is what makes it possible for you to lose weight. Although your first though may be to start exercising as much as possible, right away, you may want to refrain from doing so.

If you aren't usually physically active, it is best to start out slow. This should significantly reduce your risk of injuries.

Another one of the many ways that you may be able to achieve fasts weight loss or rapid weight loss is with the use of a cleanser. These cleanses are commonly referred to as colon cleanses or weight loss cleanses. Cleanses work by removing toxins and extra weight, actually waste, from your body. It has been said that most individuals have at least seven or eight pounds of waste stored in their bodies. A weight loss cleanse or a colon cleanse should help remove those toxins from your body.

Should you decide to try a colon cleanse or a weight loss cleanse, to help you achieve a fast weight loss, it is important that you read all directions given to you.

Some cleanses have a strict diet that you must follow. For the fastest weight loss, you may want to examine liquid cleanses, instead of those in pill formats, as they often produce the quickest results.

The above mentioned fast weight loss tips may help you achieve fast weight loss, even if it is only a small weight loss. As a reminder, it is important to proceed with caution. While it is more than possible for you to achieve your fast weight loss goal, it can also be dangerous to you and your health.

How to Find a Local Weight Loss Center

Are you looking to lose weight? If you are, have you ever thought about joining a weight loss center? A weight loss center membership is a nice way to help you achieve your goal of losing weight. If you have never been a member of a weight loss center before, you may be wondering how you can go about finding a weight loss center to join.

Before examining how you can go about finding a weight loss center to join, it is first important to know what weight loss centers are. When examining weight loss centers, you will find that weight loss centers come in a number of different formats.

Most commonly, weight loss centers are used to describe local weight loss programs, where you attend group meetings at the "center." There are some weight loss centers that have weekly or biweekly meetings, like for weigh-ins.

There are also weight loss centers where your membership fees give you access to onsite exercise equipment or the ability to attend an aerobics class.

Now that you know exactly what weight loss centers are, you are better prepared to go about finding one to join. One of the many ways that you can go about finding a weight loss center to become a member at is by using your local phone book.

When using your local phone book, you will want to check out the business directory section, which is also commonly referred to as the yellow pages.

You may be able to find the names, addresses, and telephone numbers of local weight loss centers by looking under the headings of "weight loss," or "health and fitness."

In addition to using your local phone book, you can also use the internet to help you find a local weight loss center to join. When using the internet, you can use online business directories or online phone books. These online resources are nice, but they are similar to what you would find in your local phone book.

Often times, you only get the name, address, and telephone number of a weight loss center. If you were to use an online business directory, you may also get the address to an online website, if the weight loss center in question has one.

In keeping with using the internet to help you find a local weight loss center, you can also use standard internet searches to your advantage. When performing a standard internet search, you may want to search with phrases like "weight loss centers," or "weight loss programs."

This generalized search may return results for nationally operated weight loss centers. If you are looking for a local center, you may want to incorporate your city or your state into your standard internet search as well.

Another great way that you can go about finding a local weight loss center to join is by asking those that you know for recommendations. This includes your friends, family members, coworkers, neighbors, or your doctors.

Whether the individual in question was or still is a member of the weight loss center in question or they know someone who was, you may be able to get a lot of information by speaking to those that you know.

It is also nice, as you often don't just get the name, address, or telephone number of a local weight loss center; you also should get personal recommendations and constructive criticism as well.

The above mentioned approaches are just a few of the many ways that you can go about finding local weight loss centers to join.

Although it is nice to hear recommendations from those that you know or use the internet to help you familiarize yourself with all of your options, it is important that you take the time to find the perfect weight loss center for you and needs.

This should involve examining the membership features that you have access to, the cost of becoming a member, and so forth.

How to Find the Best Weight Loss Program for You

Are you looking to lose weight? If you are, you may be interested in joining a weight loss program. When it comes to joining a weight loss program, you will find that you have a number of different options.

If this is your first time joining a weight loss program, you may be unsure as to what you should look for in a weight loss program. If that is the case, you will want to continue reading on.

One of the best ways to go about finding the perfect weight loss program for you is to ask yourself a number of important questions. One of the first questions that you should ask yourself is how much time you have to devote to weight loss meetings. If you were to join a local weight loss program, you would likely be required to attend weekly meeting.

Whether you are busy with your family or busy at work, you may not have the time to do so. In that case, you should look into joining an online weight loss program, as they are often designed for those with busy schedules.

Another question that you will want to ask yourself, when looking to find the perfect weight loss program is your willpower. Should you join an online weight loss program, you will be given more freedom, as you do not have to physically report to meetings and answer to group leaders.

While this freedom is nice, it has allowed many hopeful individuals to go off track. If you do not think that you can stick with your online weight loss program goals and instructions, it may be better to join a local weight loss program instead.

Another one of the many questions that you will want to ask yourself, when looking for a weight loss program to join, is how much money you have to spend. While it is possible to find free weight loss programs, both locally or online, it is actually quite rare.

In your search for weight loss programs, you will find that they have a wide range of membership fees.

Commonly, you will find that online weight loss programs are cheaper than locally operated weight loss programs. If you are on a budget, the cost of each weight loss program that you come across should play a large role in your decision.

You should also ask yourself if you are embarrassed with your current weight or your physical appearance. Although you should have nothing to be ashamed of, you may still feel that way.

If that is the case, you may be afraid of attending local weight loss meetings. Of course, you need to remember that everyone else in your meetings is likely feeling the same way, but you don't have to put yourself in an awkward situation.

If you are concerned with your appearance or what others may think of you, you may want to look into joining an online weight loss program instead.

The above mentioned questions are just a few of the many that you should ask yourself if you are interested in joining a weight loss program. While there are a number of benefits to joining a locally operated weight loss program, as well as an online weight loss program, you need to make the decision that is best for you and your own needs.

Is Weight Loss Surgery Your Best Option?

Are you looking to lose weight? If you are, there is a good chance that you have heard of weight loss surgery before. Weight loss surgery is how many individuals lose weight. Although weight loss surgery has helped thousands of Americans lose weight, improve their appearance, and improve their health, weight loss surgery may not be for you.

When it comes to determining if weight loss surgery is right for you, there are a number of factors that you will need to take into consideration. One of those factors is your current weight.

Most of the time, you will find that weight loss surgeons require their patients to be at least eighty pounds overweight. If you are not as overweight as recommend, you may not even be able to undergo a weight loss surgery.

If that is the case, you should keep in mind that there are a number of different weight loss approaches that you can take.

Speaking of alternative weight loss methods, have you tried any other approaches? Many individuals are able to successfully lose weight with healthy eating, exercise, and weight loss products, like diet pills.

While there are some individuals who opt for weight loss surgery right away, there are others who only use it as a last resort.

Although weight loss surgery, like gastric bypass surgery or lap-band surgery, is more than worth it, you may be able to lose your excess weight without having to spend a large amount of money doing so.

Another factor that you should take into consideration, when determining if weight loss surgery is right for you, is your health.

If you are overweight, have you been noticing any other health problems or has your doctor outlined the importance of losing weight for your health? If this has happened, you may not have a choice when it comes to undergoing weight loss surgery. For some individuals, weight loss surgery is, literally, lifesaving.

As it was previously mentioned, two popular weight loss surgeries include gastric bypass surgery and lap-band surgery. While there additional weight loss surgeries that you can undergo, these two are the most popular ones.

The surgery that you would like to undergo is also important when determining whether or not weight loss surgery is your best option.

For instance, gastric bypass surgery requires the stapling of the stomach, whereas lap-band surgery involves an adjustable or removable band.

When deciding which weight loss surgery you should undergo, your decision will need to be made in conjunction with a healthcare professional.

When examining weight loss surgeries, you will find that most surgeries reduce the stomach pouch size. For that reason, your ability to follow all instructions given to you is important.

After undergoing a weight loss surgery, like lap-band surgery or gastric bypass surgery, your healthcare professional will likely request that you develop yourself an exercise plan, as well as eat healthy.

It is important that you follow all advice given to you. With weight loss surgeries that involve the reduction of the stomach pouch, an over consumption of food can be harmful to your weight loss, as well as dangerous to your health.

The above mentioned factors are factors that may help you determine whether or not weight loss surgery is right for you.

As a reminder, it is important to remember that weight loss surgery is not your only option, when looking to lose weight, but it is a method that you should explore.

Online Weight Loss Programs: Are They Worth the Money?

Have you ever heard of an online weight loss program before? Online weight loss programs are designed to assist individuals, possibly just like you, who want to lose weight.

What it nice about online weight loss programs is that they are operated online, which is nice for those who have busy schedules; schedules that may not allow them to join locally operated weight loss programs.

If you have never joined an online weight loss program before, you may be wondering if one is right for you. Better yet, you may be wondering if an online weight loss program is worth the cost.

In all honestly, you will typically find that online weight loss programs are well worth their costs, but it all depends.

To ensure that your money is wisely spent, you will want to make sure that you choose the online weight loss program that is perfect for you and your needs.

When finding an online weight loss program that is more than worth the costs, you will want to examine the features that you have access to. Features are also commonly referred to as membership benefits or membership perks.

The program features that you have access to plays a large part in determining whether or not the online weight loss program that you want to join is worth the money.

A few of the many online weight loss features or member perks that you will want access to are outlined below.

One of the many features or membership benefits that would make an online weight loss program well worth the cost is that of healthy eating tips. As you likely already know, healthy eating is an important part of any weight loss plan.

Many online weight loss programs have healthy eating sections that include making recipes for foods and drinks, as well as shopping tips and much more.

As previously stated, healthy eating is an important part of losing weight; therefore, you should look for an online weight loss program that does have a healthy eating or a healthy foods section.

Another feature that would make an online weight loss program more than worth the costs is that of an exercise program. It has been said that exercise and healthy eating are the two most important components of losing weight. You should be able to find an online weight loss program that has an exercise section for you to access. This section may outline workouts that you should try, which may be accompanied by pictures, videos, or at least detailed directions.

You may also find charts that outline how many calories are burned with common exercises, and much more.

One feature that you may not necessarily think of, but one that is important, is that of an online message board or a community section. Community sections are often comprised of online message boards.

These sections often allow you to communicate with other online weight loss program members or group leaders.

This communication is nice as it may help to give you motivation. You may even find an online weight loss buddy or partner to help you on your journey.

Guaranteed results or free trial periods are another sign that an online weight loss program may be worth the money. Often times, many individuals are unsure as to whether or not they should pay to join an online weight loss program, as they do not know for sure that they will lose weight.

A large number of online weight loss programs give you the ability to test out their programs free of charge and then there are others that give you guaranteed results. With guarantees like these, online weight loss programs are more than worth their costs.

The above mentioned points are just a few of the many that may be able to help you decide whether or not joining an online weight loss program is worth the cost.

If you are able to find an online weight loss program with a free trial period or even just one with affordable membership rates, you may want to think about giving it a shot.

Online Weight Loss Programs: How They Work

If you are interested in losing weight, you may have thought about joining a local weight loss program or visiting a local weight loss center. Unfortunately, if you are like many other individuals who are interested in losing weight, you may not necessarily have the time to do so.

Whether you have a demanding job, a family to take care of, or both, you may find it impossible to meet up with a local weight loss group on a regular basis.

If that is the case, you may be thinking that achieving your weight loss goal is simply out of reach, but it doesn't have to be.

What many individuals do not know is that they can join an online weight loss program. Online weight loss programs are similar to many locally operated weight loss programs.

Often times, the only difference is that you do not get to meet with group leaders or other members in person. If you are searching for a way to incorporate weight loss into your busy schedule, you are urged to examine online weight loss programs. These online weight loss programs are designed for all individuals, but they are perfect for those who regularly find themselves pressed for time.

When it comes to online weight loss programs, you will find that these online weight loss programs come in a number of different formats.

For starters, it is possible to find free online weight loss programs; however, you will likely find that the best ones require the paying of a membership fee.

Although each weight loss program is likely to vary, many have affordable monthly membership rates, some as low as five dollars a month. It is also possible to find weight loss programs that are designed for women, men, those over the age of fifty, and so forth.

If you have never joined an online weight loss program before, you may be wondering a little bit more about how they work. As previously stated, not all online weight loss programs are the same.

With that in mind, however, you will find that many operate in similar matters. A few of the many member perks that you may get, when joining an online weight loss program, are outlined below.

One of the many perks or benefits to joining an online weight loss program is that you should get access to work out or exercise information.

Many online weight loss programs will give you access to their website, which should have exercises and workouts outlined for you. You should be able to get detailed directions for those exercises, pictures, and possibly even sample videos. Some more expensive online weight loss programs will give you access to customize workouts, ones which focus on the areas of your body that you would most like to improve.

Another member perk or feature that you should get access to with an online weight loss program is that of healthy recipes. Healthy eating is an important part of weight loss.

That is why many online weight loss programs have a healthy eating section. Not only may you get healthy food recipes, but you may also get moneysaving coupons, as well as cooking and food shopping tips.

As previously stated, often times the only difference between a locally operated weight loss program and an online program is the fact that you do not get to meet with the group leaders or other group members in person.

With online weight loss programs, you may not get in-person contact, but you may still be able to communicate.

Many online weight loss programs have online message boards for their members to communicate with each other.

As a reminder, it is important to remember that not all online weight loss programs are the same. Despite the possibility of a variance, you should find that most online weight loss programs are more than worth your money, especially if you regularly find yourself pressed for time.

Paying for a Weight Loss Program versus Developing Your Own

Are you interested in losing weight? Whether you would like to improve your health, improve you appearance, or do both, you may be interested in finding a weight loss plan to use.

When it comes to weight loss plans, you will find that you have a number of different options. Two of your most common options include paying for a weight loss plan or developing your own.

If this is your first time attempting to "seriously," lose weight, you may be wondering whether you should develop your own weight loss plan, also commonly referred to as a weight loss program, or pay for one.

One of the best ways to determine which weight loss plan you should use is to examine the pros and cons of each.

A few of the most influential advantages and disadvantages to developing your own weight loss plan, as well as paying for one are outlined below.

When it comes to paying for a weight loss plan or a weight loss program, you will find that you can do so locally or online. If you choose to participate in a local weight loss program or plan, you will likely meet in a centralized location.

Many times, you just get together every week or two. There are some weight loss programs where you can exercise onsite though. Should you choose to join an online weight loss program, you will likely have online meetings or discussions with trainers or other weight loss program members, either on a message board or through emails. You should also have access to healthy recipes and easy to do exercises.

One of the many advantages to paying for a weight loss program or a weight loss plan is that you are often given a professional plan. Many times, the individuals or trainers in charge of running these programs have training or firsthand experience with losing weight. This often eliminates trial and error, as many have already learned what works and what does not work with weight loss.

In all honestly, the only downside to paying to join a weight loss program or a weight loss plan is that you have to pay to do so. With that in mind, however, you should be able to find affordable weight loss programs and plans, both locally and online.

Although it is not guaranteed, many people find the most affordable help in the form of online weight loss programs or online weight loss plans.

As for developing your own weight loss plan, there are a number of advantages to doing so. One of those advantages is that you can customize your weight loss plan and program to you.

For example, if you were allergic to milk, you could work your allergy into your weight loss program, where as a paid weight loss plan or program may not do so. You can also customize your workouts to yourself. This is great if you are obese and unable to follow many workout videos, which seem like they are designed for those who already in "perfect," shape.

Another one of the many advantages to developing your own weight loss plan to follow is that it is fun to do. You also have a number of tools at your fingertips.

There are a number of websites and magazines that you can get weight loss information from; information that you can use to create your own weight loss plan to follow.

Some individuals have said that creating their own weight loss plan to follow makes them more excited about the process and more likely to see the plan all the way through.

The above mentioned factors are just a few of the many that you may want to take into consideration, when trying to determine whether you should develop your own weight loss program or join a paid weight loss program.

Many individuals have reported starting their own weight loss program and then later joining a paid one if they didn't get the results that they were hoping for.

Should You Join an Online Weight Loss Program?

Have you ever heard of an online weight loss program before? If this is your first time hearing about an online weight loss program, you may be wondering whether or not you should join one. If you are, you will want to continue reading on.

Perhaps, the biggest sign that you should think about joining an online weight loss program is if you are looking to lose weight. Whether you are interesting in improving your appearance, improving your health, or doing both, weight loss can be a stressful time.

Many weight loss programs assist you by having a daily food or exercise log for you to fill out. This has been known to motivate many online weight loss program members. Depending on the online weight loss program that you join, you should also get access to fun workouts and healthy recipes.

Another one of the many signs that you should think about joining an online weight loss program is if you regularly find yourself pressed on time.

Whether you have a family to take care of, a demanding job, or both, you may find it difficult to eat healthy or maintain a regular exercise program.

Joining an online weight loss program is a nice alternative to attending a local weight loss program, one that often requires you to meet for an hour or two a week.

Another one of the many signs that you should join an online weight loss program is if they are able to find an online weight loss program that is perfect for you. What is nice about online weight loss programs is that they come in a number of different formats.

For instance, it is possible to find "generalized," online weight loss programs, which are designed for all different individuals. On the other hand, there are themed weight loss programs, like ones that are designed for men, women, and senior citizens.

Finding the perfect online weight loss program makes it well worth it for you to join one.

Speaking of finding the perfect online weight loss program, the best way to find one is to perform a standard internet search. When performing a standard internet search, you may want to search with phrases like "online weight loss programs," or "online weight loss plans."

If you are looking for something specific, like an online weight loss program for women, you will want to incorporate that into your standard internet search.

You can also ask those that you know for recommendations or find online discussions where online weight loss programs are being discussed.

When searching for an online weight loss program, you will likely come across multiple programs that may interest you. When it comes to choosing an online weight loss program to join, it is advised that you take the features that you have access to, like online message board communication and healthy recipes, as well as costs into consideration. An online weight loss program that has more features or online resources for you may be worth paying a little bit more money for.

If you fit the above mentioned criteria, you may want to look into joining an online weight loss program. In fact, you may even find an online weight loss program that gives you a free trial period.

This is the perfect opportunity to determine whether or not an online weight loss program is right for you.

The Dangers of Rapid Weight Loss

Are you interested in losing weight? If you are, are you looking for a rapid weight loss? Rapid weight loss, also commonly referred to as quick weight loss or fast weight loss, involves losing weight in a short period of time, often anywhere from two to seven days.

Each year, in the United States, hundreds of thousands of Americans are interested in rapidly losing weight. Many people wish to lose weight before an important event, like an upcoming vacation or a wedding.

While it is defiantly possible to understand how you can want to lose weight quickly, namely as fast as possible, you need to proceed with caution. Although it is possible to lose weight, at least a little bit of it, in a relatively quick period of time, you should know that there are dangers associated with doing so.

One of the many dangers of rapid weight loss is some of the many measures that some people take. For instance, it is common to hear of individuals who have decided not to eat, while trying to achieve a rapid weight loss.

Going without food, for even a short period of time, can be dangerous to your health. A better alternative is to cut back on the food that you do eat or to just make sure that it is healthy foods in which you are eating.

By limiting your calories, you should be able to achieve at least a small weight loss in the time that you were looking to. It is just very important that you do eat.

In addition to eating healthy, another component of weight loss is exercise. Unfortunately, many individuals do not realize that it can take up to one week to notice the signs of exercise. With that in mind, the more weight you need to lose, the sooner it is that you may start seeing results.

While exercise is a major component of losing weight, it is important that you do not overdo it, especially if you haven't had a regular exercise plan. Running on the treadmill for three hours, instead of thirty minutes, may help reduce your calorie intake, but, at the same time, it may also land you in the hospital.

Another problem that is often associated with rapid weight loss is the taking of medications or other weight loss products.

The good news is that many of these products do work and some are even safe, but you may not be able to tell what you are getting.

If you are interested in using a weight loss product, like a diet pill or a cleanser, to help you lose weight, it is important that you do the proper amount of research first.

This research may involve checking product reviews, to see if the product is effective, or speaking with a healthcare professional.

As you can see, it is important that you proceed with caution when trying to achieve rapid weight loss. Although unexpected events or appearances do popup, most individuals have at least a months' worth of notice before attending a large event, like a wedding or even a vacation.

As soon as you know about your upcoming event, you are advised to start trying to lose weight then, if you are interested in doing so. Rapid weight loss can be dangerous; therefore, you shouldn't rely on it if possible.

Using the Internet to Develop Your Own Weight Loss Plan

Are you interested in developing your own weight loss plan? If you are looking to lose weight, there is a good chance that you may be interested in doing so. Although you can pay to have a weight loss plan supplied to you or you can choose to join an existing weight loss program, you may find the cost of doing so a little bit difficult, especially if you are on a budget. That is why many choose to develop their own weight loss plans.

If this is your first time developing a weight loss plan for yourself, you may not necessarily know how you should proceed. What is nice about developing a weight loss plan for yourself is that you have freedom.

With that in mind, you will still want to make sure that your weight loss plan is one that you can benefit from and one that you can lose weight while on.

For that reason, you may want to think about turning to the internet, when looking to develop your own weight loss plan or weight loss program.

When it comes to using the internet to help you develop your own weight loss plan, there are a number of different ways that the internet can offer your assistance.

For starters, a good part of a weight loss program involves eating healthy. For many individuals, eating healthy is something that is difficult to do, as they are unsure as to what they should cook or how they should cook it.

There are a number of websites that you can find online, many of which are free to use, that give you access to healthy foods and recipes. Many of these recipes are accompanied by pictures; therefore, you should be able to tell right away whether or not the food in question is something that you would eat.

Another part of losing weight involves exercise. For some individuals, taking a simple walk is enough to help them lose weight, but others must participate in more active exercise activities.

If you are one of those individuals, you can find a number of websites that outline exercises that you should be able to do. You will likely find a number of fitness websites that come with detailed pictures or videos, which outline each step of the workout in question.

You can also use the internet to order weight loss resources, like weight loss books or exercise equipment. One piece of exercise equipment that you may want to look into buy is that of an exercise video.

What is nice about using the internet to find an exercise video, which you can incorporate into your at-home weight loss program is, that you can not only buy videos online, but you can also find product reviews.

Product reviews are a great way to determine if the exercise video you are interested in buying is really worth the money.

Once you have found a number of exercises that you would like to do or a number of healthy meals that you would like to make for yourself, you are advised to develop yourself a list, in writing or on the computer.

This list can act as a schedule for you. For instance, you could outline each workout that you would like to do on Monday's, as well as which meals you would like to eat on that same day. Having a detailed weight loss plan for each day of the week is likely to improve the chances of you following your own plan.

As you can see, the internet is a nice tool to have, when looking to create your own weight loss plan. For the best results, with finding what you need online, you may want to perform a standard internet search.

As a reminder, not everyone is able to develop their own at-home weight loss plans and follow them.

If you find that you are having a difficult time with staying on track, you may want to think about joining one of your local weight loss programs or even an online weight loss program.

Weight Loss Centers: What Are They and Should You Use Them?

Have you recently decided that you would like to lose weight? If you have, you will find that you have a number of different options.

For instance, you can casually decide to lose weight, develop your own structured weight loss program, join an online weight loss program, or you can become a member of a local weight loss center.

Although each weight loss method is effective, you may be interested in joining a weight loss center.

If you have never been a member of a weight loss center before, you may be wondering about them. Weight loss centers are often used to describe local weight loss programs.

When joining a weight loss center, you will likely attend weekly, biweekly, or monthly meetings at the "center," location.

Most weight loss centers require the payment of a monthly membership fee. Despite the possibility of a variance, these membership fees are often almost always affordable.

When looking for a weight loss center to become a member at, you should know that not all weight loss centers are the same. For instance, there are some weight loss centers that only host weekly, biweekly, or monthly meetings.

These meetings are often used to record your weight, as well as socialize and communicate with others who are looking to lose weight, just like you.

On the other hand, there are weight loss center that give you more membership benefits. These types of weight loss centers may have healthy eating cooking classes, instructional exercise classes, and a fully equipped fitness center for you to use.

If you are able to find a weight loss center that has an onsite fitness center or instructional classes, whether they be for eating or exercising, you are urged to further examine the weight loss center.

Yes, the membership fees for these types of weight loss centers may be a little bit higher, but they are well worth it. In fact, those who join weight loss centers that have instructional classes or onsite gyms often report better results. This is because you often feel more motivated to exercise and eat healthy and you also get support from other hopeful weight loss losers at the same time as well.

If you are interested in joining a weight loss center, the first thing that you should do is familiarize yourself with all of your options.

This may include asking those that you know, like friends, family members, coworkers, neighbors, or your doctor, for recommendations, using the internet, or your local phone book.

Once you have the contact information for a number of local weight loss centers, you can do a little bit of research or comparison.

What you will want to do is examine all of the membership benefits that you are given, like access to healthy recipes, food journals, access to an onsite gym, and so forth. Then, you will want to compare membership fees.

If you live in a larger city or town, there is a good chance that you will find at least two weight loss centers for you to join. That is why it is important that you take the time to examine and compare all of your options.

Yes, any weight loss center is better than no weight loss center, but you should take the time to find the weight loss center that is the perfect match for you and your own personal needs.

Doing so may result in you achieving your weight loss goal and in a fun and exciting way.

Weight Loss Exercise Products You May Want to Buy

Are you interested in losing weight and improving your appearance? If you are, you should know the importance of exercise. Exercise burns off calories, which reduces your calorie intake, which, in turn, makes it possible for you to lose weight.

If this is the first time that you have decided to seriously try to lose weight, you may be looking to buy exercise equipment for yourself. If you are, you will want to continue reading on. Below, a few popular pieces of exercise equipment that you may look into buying are outlined.

One piece of exercise equipment that you may want to look into buying is that of a treadmill. Treadmills are, perhaps, the most well-known piece of exercise equipment available.

What is nice about treadmills is that they come in a number of different styles. For instance, you can find treadmills that are powered by electricity and then treadmills that are powdered by your own walking.

This is nice as it often results in treadmills being available for a wide range of prices. Whether you have one hundred dollars to spend on a treadmill or one thousand dollars, you should be able to find a treadmill for your home weight loss plan.

Another piece of exercise equipment that you may want to look into buying, for your at-home weight loss plan, is that of an elliptical machine.

Elliptical machines are nice, as they often combine multiple exercises. More advanced elliptical machines, also commonly referred to as deluxe elliptical machines, often given you an upper body workout and a lower body workout as well.

Elliptical machines are often referred to as combination stair climbers and ski machines.

An exercise bike is another popular piece of exercise equipment that you may want to think about buying for your at-home weight loss program. Like an elliptical machine, there are many exercise bikes that give you an upper body and a lower body workout.

These are points to take into consideration, should you decide to buy an exercise bike for yourself. Like treadmills, exercise bikes come in a number of different formats and styles; therefore, they are sold for a wide range of prices.

One piece of exercise equipment that you may not necessarily think about buying, but one that you should examine is that of a trampoline. When it comes to trampolines, you will find that they come in a number of different formats.

For instance, it is possible to find larger size trampolines, ones that are ideal for backyards and often associated with recreational play. While these trampolines can also be used for exercise, there are smaller, mini trampolines that are designed for exercises, as well as indoor use. These types of trampolines are often fun, exciting, and affordable.

The above mentioned pieces of exercise equipment are ones that are often larger in size and occasionally more expensive. If you are looking for more affordable pieces of exercise equipment or more compact pieces, you still have an unlimited number of products to choose from.

For instance, there are yoga and Pilates items that are often affordable and small in size. Exercise balls and resistance bands are popular items that you may want to take the time to examine.

There are also weight sets that you can buy or you can buy a few individuals weights to use at home. When it comes to exercising at home, your options are, literally, unlimited.

When it comes to buying exercise equipment for yourself, you will find that you have a number of different options. You can shop locally or online. Exercise equipment is sold at sports stores, as well as traditional department stores.

If you are on a budget, you may want to look into buying used exercise equipment. Used exercise equipment can often be found on online auction websites, in thrift stores, and at yard sales.

As outlined above, there are a number of different exercise equipment pieces that you can use to help you lose weight at home. Whether you choose to buy some of the pieces outlined above or something else, you are sure to have a fun and exciting time working to achieve your weight loss goal.

Weight Loss Pills: Should You Use Them?

Have you been trying to lose weight with the use of exercise and healthy eating? If you have, have you still been coming up short on your weight loss goal?

If you have, you may be interested in seeking help through the use of weight loss products, namely weight loss pills. Although you may be thinking about giving weight loss pills a chance, you may be wondering if you should.

When it comes to determining whether or not weight loss pills are right for you, there are a number of different questions that you will want to ask yourself.

These questions can help you truly determine if weight loss pills are right for you. A few of the many questions that you may want to ask yourself, concerning weight loss pills, are outlined below.

One of the many questions that you will want to ask yourself is if you have really tired losing weight. Losing weight "naturally," often involves exercise and healthy eating.

Have you been exercising? Exercising can involve visiting your local fitness center, putting an exercise video in your DVD player, or something as simple as taking a nightly walk. Eating healthy involves cutting all sweets from your diet or at least significantly reducing them. If you haven't taken these steps yet, you may want to first try losing weight naturally. If that doesn't work, weight loss diet pills may be something for you to consider.

Although there are a number of reasons for weight gain, one of the most common reasons involves eating too much food. If you regularly find yourself eating more food than you should or more food than you need to, why do you think that you do so?

Are you just eating because you are bored or does your body sense that you are hungry? This is important question that you need to answer, as many weight loss pills are designed to suppress your hunger.

While this can help many individuals reduce the amount of food that they eat and the number of calories they take in, it will only help you if you think that your body is telling you that you are still hungry.

If you are what is commonly referred to as a "bored eater," there is a good chance that you will still continue to eat.

Another question that you need to ask yourself is if you can afford the costs of weight loss pills. When examining the cost of weight loss pills, you will find that they are sold for a wide range of prices.

Although it is important to make sure that you can afford the cost of weight loss pills, it is important that you do not comprise quality for costs.

If you cannot afford the weight loss pills that come highly rated and recommend, you may just end up wasting your money on weight loss pills that may not necessarily work. That is why it is advised that you consult with your doctor or search for weight loss diet pill reviews online, before making any purchases.

The above mentioned questions are just a few of the many that you may want to ask yourself, before you automatically go out and buy weight loss pills for yourself.

As a reminder, it is important that you do the proper amount of research before you buy weight loss pills, should you decide to do so. Weight loss diet pills are not all created equally; therefore, they have varying results.

Weight Loss Surgery: Is It Worth the Money?

Are you interested in losing weight? If you are, how much weight would you like to lose? If you are looking to lose eighty pounds or more in weight, did you know that you may be a candidate for weight loss surgery?

Although it is nice to hear that you may be a candidate for weight loss surgery, you may be wondering if weight loss surgery is right for you. More importantly, you may be wondering if weight loss surgery is worth the money. If that is a question that you would like the answer, to you will want to continue reading on.

In short, the question as to whether or not weight loss surgery is worth the money has a simple answer; it all depends. While that may not have necessarily been the answer that you were looking for, it is the truth.

For many individuals, weight loss surgery is well worth it; however, there are others who don't end up benefiting from weight loss surgery.

To determine if weight loss surgery is worth the cost to you, personally, you will want to take a number of factors into consideration.

One of the many factors that you will want to take into consideration, when determining if weight loss surgery is worth the cost for you, is your weight.

You will find that many weight loss surgeons require that you are at least eighty pounds overweight to undergo weight loss surgery. With that in mind, you may be able to find a surgeon who will make an exception, but that doesn't necessarily mean that you should opt for surgery.

If you are able to try to lose the weight on your own, through the use of exercise, eating healthy, or diet pills, you may find it more affordable to do so.

Your health is another factor that you should take into consideration, when trying to determine if weight loss surgery is right for you. Weight loss surgery is commonly referred to as a lifesaving medical procedure. Those who are severely obese put their health at risk and may experience an early death. If you are severely obese, your physician may recommend weight loss surgery. If that is the case, weight loss surgery is more than worth the costs, as you cannot put a price tag on your health and wellbeing.

Your ability to set goals and stay with them is another factor to consider, when determining if weight loss surgery is worth the cost to you. Weight loss surgery may help you lose weight right away, but the surgery alone will not help you lose weight.

With a reduced stomach pouch, which is how most weight loss surgeries work, you must limit the amount of food that you eat. If you do not do so, you may gain your weight back and possibly endanger your health.

If you do not think that you can follow all of the instructions given to you, following a weight loss surgery, surgery may not be the best option for you.

The above mentioned factors are just a few of the many that can help you decide if weight loss surgery is right for you or if it is worth the cost. As a reminder, it is important that you take the time to first consult with your doctor. Not all individuals are candidates for weight loss surgery.

Weight Loss: Why Exercise Is Important

Are you interested in losing weight? If you are, you may be in the process of developing a weight loss plan for yourself. For many individuals, a weight loss plan is a guide that they can follow and one that may help to give them motivation.

If this is your first time developing a weight loss plan for yourself, it is important that you place a focus on exercise, as exercise is important component of weight loss.

Although it is nice to hear that exercise is an important part of a weight loss plan, you may be wondering exactly why that is. For your body to lose weight, you must see a reduction in your calorie intake.

The amount of calories that you need to reduce, in order to lose weight, will all depend on your current weight and your hopeful weight loss goal.

Unfortunately, this is where many individuals automatically assume that they can't eat three meals a day and many actually just stop eating. This is not only dangerous to your health, but it can be deadly.

Instead of reducing your calorie intake by solely limiting the amount of foods that you eat, you can use exercise to your advantage. By exercising, you burn off calories.

These are calories in which your body can use to help you lose weight. If you have a specific weight loss goal, like one that involves losing at least twenty pounds, you may want to focus on fun exercises or workouts, but also ones that burn the most calories. Adding exercise to your weight loss plan is a natural and a healthy way to lose weight.

Since it is important to incorporate to exercise into your weight loss plan, you may be wondering how you can go about doing so. In all honestly, there are an unlimited number of ways that you can go about using exercise to help you lose weight.

For starters, you can buy a collection, even just a small collection, of exercise equipment. Exercise equipment can include items such as exercise balls, weights, a treadmill, a stair climber, and so forth.

Even if you have limited financial resources, you should be able to find a number of exercise equipment pieces that are within your budget.

Although you should be able to find a number of exercise equipment pieces, including instructional workout DVDs, for affordable prices, you may be looking to limit your weight loss plan investments.

If that is the case, you may want to take the time to examine your local gyms or fitness clubs. While some fitness clubs and gyms have relatively high membership fees, you can also find a number of them with affordable membership rates.

It is also important to mention that many fitness clubs and gyms are open accommodating hours, often making it easy to exercise before work, after work, or even during a lunch break of yours.

Despite the fact that exercise is often associated with exercise equipment, like a treadmill, that is not all that exercise is about. Exercise can also involve something simple like going for a walk or taking the stairs instead of the elevator at work.

If you would prefer to exercise, for free, in your spare time, you may want to consider finding an exercise buddy. This is a person who can work out with you, even if it just involves walking around your local shopping mall.

Not only can you make a new friend or strengthen your relationship with one of your current friends, having an exercise buddy or an exercise partners often means that you are more likely to stick with your weight loss plan and achieve your weight loss goals.

As outlined above, it is extremely important that you incorporate exercise into your weight loss plan, especially if you are serious about losing weight and wish to do so in a healthy matter. With multiple ways to go about incorporating exercise into your weight loss plan, there really isn't any excuse for not doing so.

What to Consider Before Buying Weight Loss Pills

Are you looking to lose weight? If you are like many other individuals who are hoping to lose weight, there is a good chance that you may turn to weight loss pills, also commonly referred to as diet pills.

Although weight loss pills are a great way to help you lose weight, you need to be cautious when using them.

If this is your first time attempting to use weight loss pills, also commonly referred to as diet pills, to help you lose weight, there are a number of important factors that you should first take into consideration.

These factors may help to make it easier, as well as safer, for you to find and buy weight loss pills. Here are just a few of the many factors that you should take into consideration, when looking to buy weight loss pills, are outlined below.

One of the many things that you need to take into consideration, when looking to buy weight loss pills is that of cost. Weight loss pills, as you will soon find out, are sold in a wide range of different prices.

It is common to find weight loss pills that sell for as low as twenty dollars, but others that can sell for three or even four hundred dollars. It is important that you find a weight loss pill that you can afford to buy.

If you cannot afford the cost of weight loss pills, you may want to examine more "natural," ways to lose weight.

The manufacturer of the weight loss pill in question is another factor that you should take into consideration. The manufacturer in question and their history can give you great insight into a weight loss pill, like if it is one that truly works or not.

If a company regularly has a bad reputation of selling weight loss pills that do not work, there is a good chance that you should stay away from that manufacturer and all of their products. Although weight loss pills are often associated with poor results, it is also important to remember that the wrong weight loss pills may also put your health at risk.

In conjunction with examining the reputation or history of the weight loss pill manufacturer in question, you are also advised to examine all of the weight loss pills that you would like to try.

As previously mentioned, there are many weight loss pills that work great and others that do not work at all. To save yourself time and money, you will want to try and find the weight loss pills that have been proven successful.

One of the best ways to go about doing so is by visiting online weight loss websites or message boards, reading product reviews, or by first consulting with a healthcare professional.

It is also important that you first examine the ingredients in a weight loss pill before you make your final purchase. Most importantly, it is important to determine whether or not you are allergic to any of the ingredients.

It is also important to see if any of the ingredients in your preferred weight loss pill are dangerous or if they have been recalled. The best ways to find out this information is by consulting with a healthcare professional or by performing a standard internet search.

You may want to perform an individual standard internet search with the name of each ingredient.

Another factor that you should take into consideration, when looking to buy weight loss pills is your point of purchase. Weight loss pills are sold by a number of different retailers, both on and offline.

If you are shopping online, it is important to make sure that you are doing business with a reputable and trustworthy retailer.

If you are shopping locally, it may be a good idea to avoid buying weight loss pills from dollar stores or discount stores.

The above mentioned factors are just a few of the many factors that you will want to take into consideration, when looking to buy weight loss pills. Generally speaking, weight loss pills are a great way to help you lose weight, as long as you know exactly what you are buying.

What to Consider When Choosing an Exercise Video

Are you interested in losing weight? If you are, you may be interested in starting your own weight loss program. Of course, you can join a local weight loss program or even an online weight loss program, but many individuals prefer to do their own, at-home weight loss programs.

If you are one of those individuals, you may be interested in buying exercise videos. Exercise videos, also commonly referred to as workout videos, are a great addition to any weight loss program.

Although you may have bought workout videos before, have you even done so when seriously trying to lose weight? In the United States, a large number of individuals buy exercise videos just because.

Just because exercise videos are a lot different than exercise videos that are a part of a weight loss plan. That is why you should shop for them differently.

When it comes to buying exercise videos for yourself, as a part of your weight loss program, there are number of important factors that you may want to take into consideration.

These factors will not only make buying exercise videos for yourself easier, but they will also help to ensure that you choose the exercise video or videos that are best for you and your own personal needs.

A few of the many factors that you should take into consideration, when buying an exercise video are outlined below.

One of the many factors that you will want to take into consideration, when buying exercise videos as a part of your weight loss plan, is the type of exercises that you want to do.

For instance, you often get to choose between traditional aerobic videos, yoga, Pilates, kickboxing, and so forth. To spice up your weight loss plan and to keep it fun and exciting, you may want to think about buying a collection of exercise videos, particularly a mixture of them.

Another one of the many factors that you will want to take into consideration, when buying an exercise video for your weight loss program, is difficulty. What you need to remember is that many workout videos come in sessions.

For instance, it is possible to find kickboxing videos that are designed for beginners, those at the intermediate level, as well as those at an advanced level.

You want to make sure that you choose the right video for yourself. If you are not careful, you may end up with an advanced workout video that you cannot even use, as you are unable to keep up with the instructor.

Cost is another factor that you may want to take into consideration, when buying workout videos or exercise videos for yourself. In your search for exercise videos, you will find that they are sold for a wide range of prices.

Some are affordable, others are a little bit more costly, and many are downright expensive. Of course, the expensive workout videos may be worth the cost, but you never really know until you order them.

One way to help make sure that you are spending your money wisely is to search for exercise video reviews online. This can often be done with a standard internet search.

The above mentioned factors are just a few of the many that you may want to take into consideration, when buying exercise videos to incorporate into your at-home weight loss program. Most times, you will find that any exercise video is better than no video at all, but taking the time to find the perfect one will likely make your weight loss program much more enjoyable.

What to Consider When Choosing a Weight Loss Center

If you are interested in losing weight, you may have thought about joining a weight loss center. Weight loss centers are often used to describe weight loss programs that are locally operated.

If this is your first time looking to join a weight loss center, you may be unsure as to what you should look for in one. An important part of joining a weight loss center is finding the weight loss center that is perfect for you and your own personal needs.

For that reason, there are a number of factors, which are outlined below, that you will want to take into consideration.

One of the many factors that you will want to take into consideration, when looking for a weight loss center to join, is the location. With gas prices high, many individuals find it difficult to travel long distances.

You will have to pay money to become a member at a weight loss center; therefore, you should be careful about adding on extra costs, like the cost of gasoline, to your membership. If, at all possible, you should look for weight loss centers that are conveniently located either close to your home or your place of business.

Speaking of costs, as previously mentioned, you will have to pay to become a member of a weight loss center. This cost will vary depending on the weight loss center in question.

On average, most weight loss center memberships are around twenty or thirty dollars a month. With that in mind, it is possible to find weight loss centers that cost more money.

If you are on a budget, a weight loss center membership fee may have an impact on the weight loss center that you chose to become a member at.

Although it is important to find a weight loss center that you can afford, you don't want to have your decision be based solely on costs. You will want to take the time to examine each weight loss center that you come across.

For instance, you should be able to find some weight loss centers that only have weekly or monthly meetings or weigh-ins for members to attend.

On the other hand, there are weight loss centers that may have exercise classes or a fitness gym, which you should gain access to as a member. If you are able to find a quality weight loss center or one that comes highly rated and recommend, higher membership fees may be worth it.

When looking to find the perfect weight loss center for you and your needs, it may be a good idea to do a little bit of research. With the internet, it is easy to review a company or a program, like a weight loss program. With a standard internet search, preferably with the name of the weight loss center in question, you should be able to come across program reviews or online discussions.

Research is not only a great way to find weight loss centers that has great reviews, but it is also a great way to learn of any weight loss centers that you should avoid or ones that are known for not being worth the costs.

The above mentioned factors are just a few of the many that you will want to take into consideration, when looking to find a weight loss center to join.

Although many weight loss centers come highly rated and recommended, it is important to find the weight loss center that can best fit you and your needs.

What to Consider When Choosing a Weight Loss Cleanse

Are you interested in losing weight? If you are, have you heard of weight loss cleanses, also commonly referred to as colon cleanses, before? If you have not, you may want to take the time to examine them.

Colon cleanses are mostly used to remove unwanted toxins from the body, but they can also be used in weight loss. That is why it is sometimes possible to find colon cleanses being referred to as weight loss cleanses.

If you have never tried a colon cleanse before, namely to lose weight, you may be wondering what you should look for in a colon cleanse. If that is the case, you will want to continue reading on.

Outlined below are a few of the many points that you should take into consideration, when looking to buy a colon cleanse.

Perhaps, the most important factor to take into consideration, when looking to buy a colon cleanse or a weight loss cleanse, is safety. It is important that you find a colon cleanse that is safe to use.

Colon cleanses and weight loss cleanses are made and sold by a number of different manufacturers and distributors. While many colon and weight loss cleanses do work, you will find that not all do.

In fact, there are even some colon cleanses which can put your health at risk. That is why it is important that you review each colon or weight loss cleanse that you are interested in buying.

When it comes to researching colon cleanses and weight loss cleanses, you have a number of different options. Perhaps, the easiest way to review this popular weight loss tools is by performing a standard internet search.

You may want to perform a standard internet search with the name of the colon cleanse that you would like to try. You will want to examine all information that you come across, especially product reviews.

Another way that you can determine if the colon cleanse or weight loss cleanse that you are interested in trying is safe is by consulting with a healthcare professional, like a dietician or your primary care physician.

Another factor that you will want to take into consideration is the length of the colon cleanses or weight loss cleanse in question. When examining the length of the colon cleanse in question, you will find that it often depends on the type of cleanse that you are using.

You should be able to find colon cleanses or weight loss cleanses that are in pill format, those that are in ready-to-drink format, as well as those that can be mixed into a drink.

For the most part, you will find that drinkable colon cleanses require shorter use times, like for two or three days. It is common to find colon cleanses, especially those in the pill formats, which need to be taken for up to thirty days or more.

The directions of the colon cleanse or weight loss cleanse that you would like to try is also important when choosing a weight loss cleanse. As with the length of a colon cleanse, you will find that the directions of each cleanse also varies.

For instance, there are some colon cleanses, namely those in pill formats, that allow you to go about eating your normal diet. On the other hand, there are some colon cleanses that require you to limit your food and drink intake, often to specific products.

If you choose a colon cleanse that requires you to only eat certain foods or go without eating for a day, it is important to make sure that you can follow those directions. If not, your colon cleanse May not work as intended and you may not be able to lose weight.

The above mentioned factors are a few of the many that you should take into consideration, when looking to buy a weight loss cleanses or colons cleanse for yourself. While some colon cleanses are not marketed as weight loss products, you will find that many do result in weight loss.

You're Weight Loss Surgery Options

Are you looking to lose weight? If you are, you likely already know that you have a number of different options. For instance, you can go about losing weight naturally, with the use of exercise and healthy eating.

You can also lose weight with the assistance of weight loss products, like diet pills. Another option that you have is weight loss surgery.

Although all of the previous weight loss methods are popular, weight loss surgery is rapidly increasing in popularity.

If you are interested in undergoing weight loss surgery, you are not alone. As previously mentioned, weight loss surgery is increasing in popularity.

If you have never considered weight loss surgery before, you may be wondering what all of your options are. While there are a number of different weight loss surgical procedures that you can undergo, you will find that there are two main procedures.

These procedures, which include gastric bypass surgery and lap-band surgery, are outlined below.

Gastric bypass surgery is a weight loss surgery that involves the stapling of the stomach. That is why this procedure is also commonly referred to as stomach stapling.

When undergoing gastric bypass surgery, your surgeon will portion off some of your stomach, making a smaller pouch.

Your intestine will then be rerouted, making it so that your food consumption only impacts a portion of your stomach. This is what makes it possible for you lose weight with gastric bypass surgery.

Although gastric bypass surgery is a great weight loss surgery to undergo, it isn't right for everyone. Most physicians require their patients to be around eighty pounds or more overweight.

In some rare instances, those who are less than eighty pounds overweight are able to undergo gastric bypass surgery if their health is at risk or if they have other medical problems, such as diabetes.

As previously stated, lap-band surgery is another weight loss surgery that is increasing in popularity. Lap-band surgery is similar to gastric bypass surgery.

When undergoing lap-band surgery, your stomach pouch is made smaller. One of the few differences is that your stomach is not stapled, but an adjustable band is used.

That is one of the reasons why lap-band surgery is so popular, as the band used can be completely removed or easily adjusted.

Lap-band surgery and gastric bypass surgery are not the only weight loss surgeries available to you, but they are two of the most popular. Thousands of Americans have undergone these two weight loss surgeries.

For many individuals, weight loss surgery is a last resort. Many who undergo weight loss surgery have not had success with losing weight any other way.

If you are interested in undergoing a weight loss surgical procedure, you will want to speak with your physician.

One of the many reasons why it is important to speak with your doctor or another healthcare professional is because weight loss surgery isn't right for everyone. In addition to being at the "right," weight, you also need to have the willpower to reduce your food consumption.

If you eat too much food, namely too much food for your stomach to hold, you can not only harm your weight loss progress, but you can also put your health at risk.

That is why your weight loss surgery decision is not one that you can make alone; it is one that must be made in conjunction with a healthcare professional.

www.ingramcontent.com/pod-product-compliance
Lightning Source LLC
Chambersburg PA
CBHW070303290526
45791CB00003B/1064